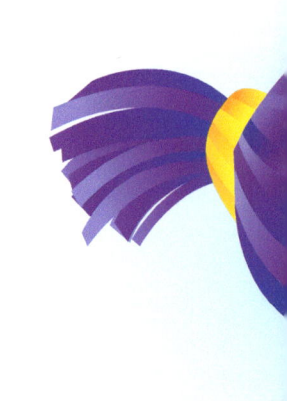

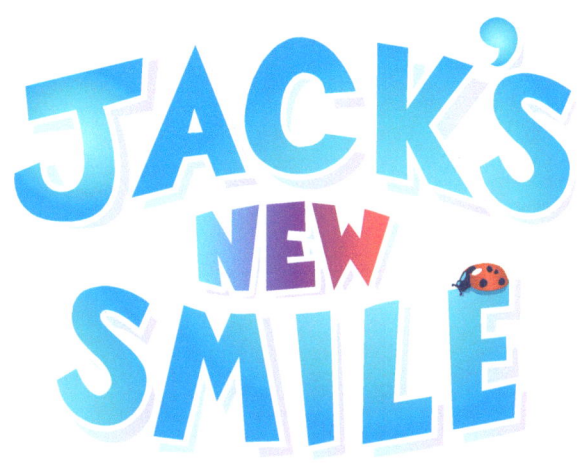

JACK'S NEW SMILE

HAVING A BABY WITH CLEFT LIP AND PALATE

WRITTEN BY
Ruth Trivelpiece, MEd
Suzanne West, MSN
Jennifer Rhodes, MD

PICTURES BY
Brooke Fetissoff

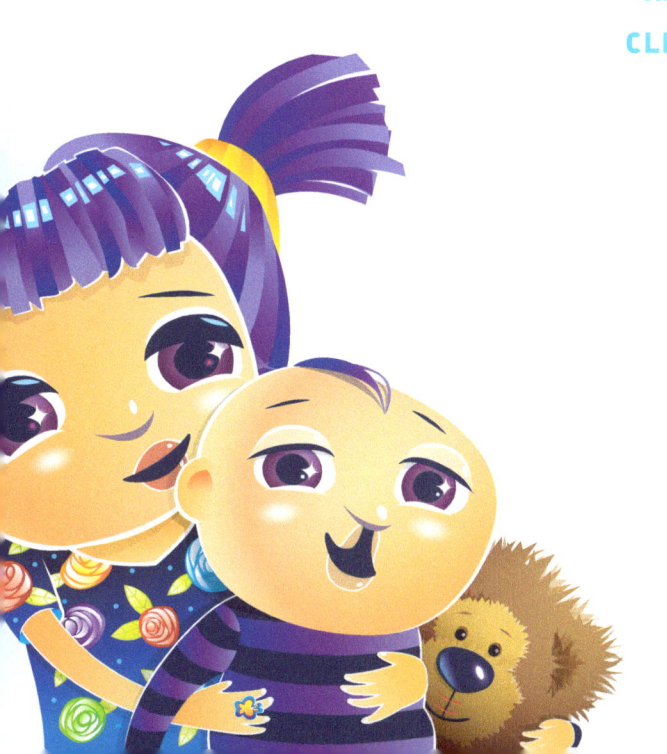

Copyright © 2017 by Ruth Trivelpiece, Suzanne West, Jennifer Rhodes, and Brooke Fetissoff.

All Rights Reserved.

DEDICATION

This book was made possible by the generous donation from Elizabeth Paull in honor of her uncle William Adolph Paull. Mr. Paull was born with a cleft lip and palate during the Great Depression. Children born at that time were not able to receive the level of care our children receive today. It is Ms. Paull's wish for all children born with a cleft to reach their full potential.

ACKNOWLEDGEMENT

We would like to thank the Children's Hospital Foundation and Children's Hospital of Richmond at Virginia Commonwealth University for the support and partnership they provide for the Center for Craniofacial Care.

Our heartfelt thanks are given to Brooke, our amazing illustrator, who constantly created beautiful pictures and inspired us with her creativity, imagination, and dedication to this book.

INTRODUCTION

This book was written for brothers and sisters of a new baby with cleft lip/palate. It is also intended for children born with a cleft to help them learn about themselves. Children may not understand why they, or the new baby in their family, have a cleft. This book is meant to provide some answers to questions children may not know how to ask.

We hope that by reading this story, your child will know that having a cleft is not scary or bad. Your family is like any other family, although you may have more doctor visits, especially the first year of life!

If your child or new baby has a cleft lip without a cleft palate, or a cleft palate alone, explain this to your child as you read the book. Feel free to use this book as a starting point for a more detailed talk with older children.

Meet my new baby brother, Jack.

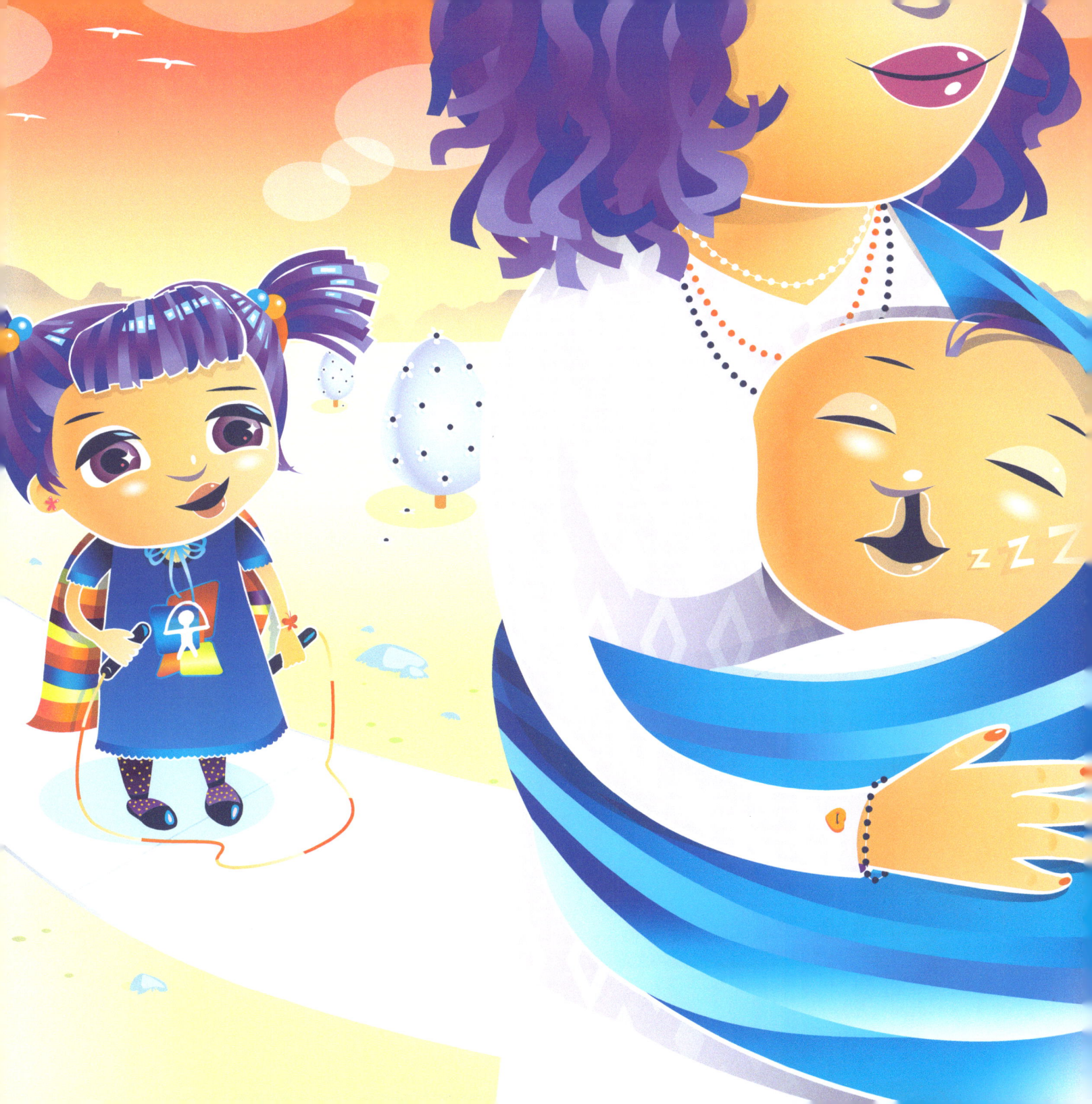

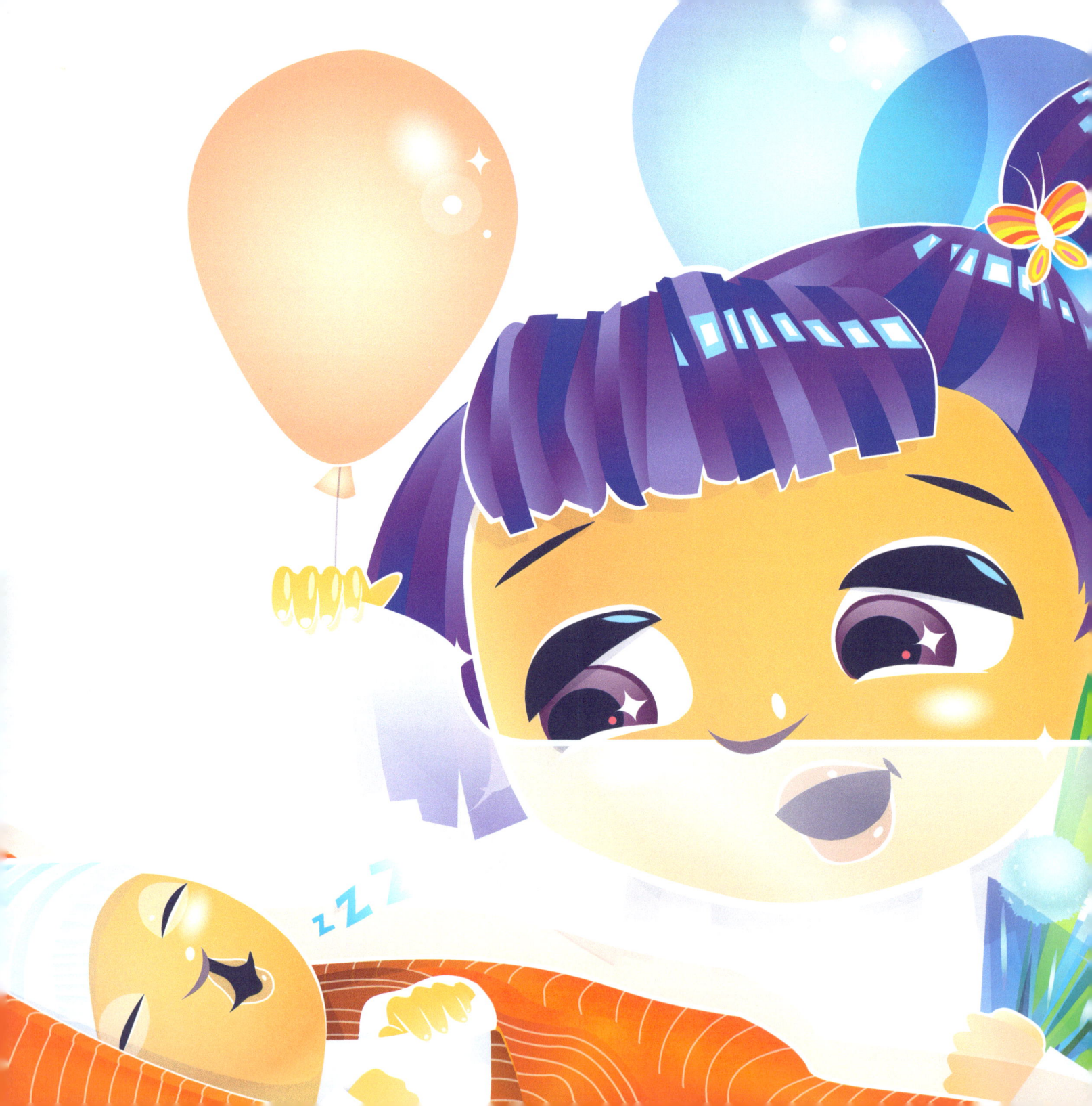

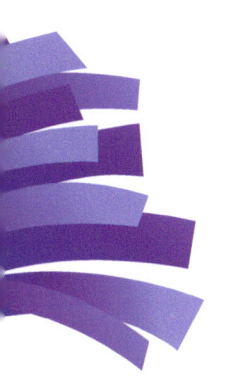

When I **first** saw him, I asked Mom...

Why does his mouth look different?

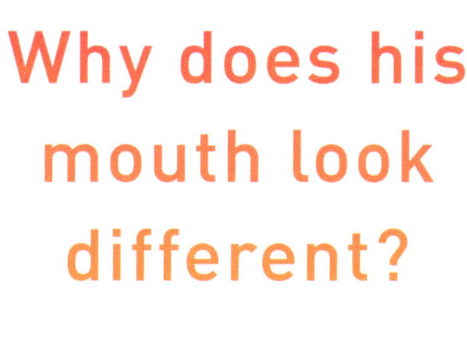

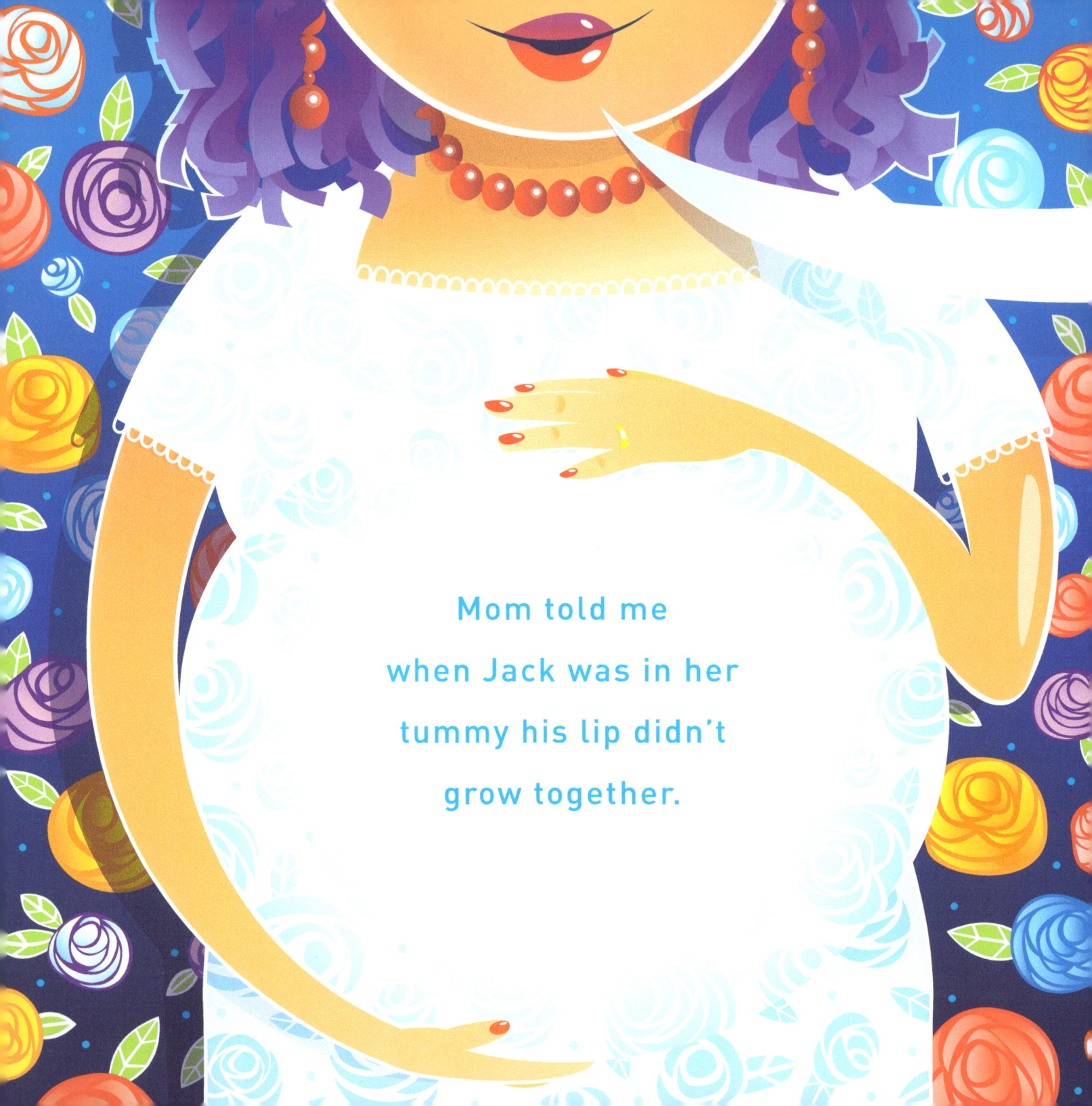

Mom told me when Jack was in her tummy his lip didn't grow together.

It's nobody's fault, sweetheart. Some babies are born this way. It's called a *cleft lip.*

If you peek in his mouth, you can see a hole on top. That's called a *cleft palate*.

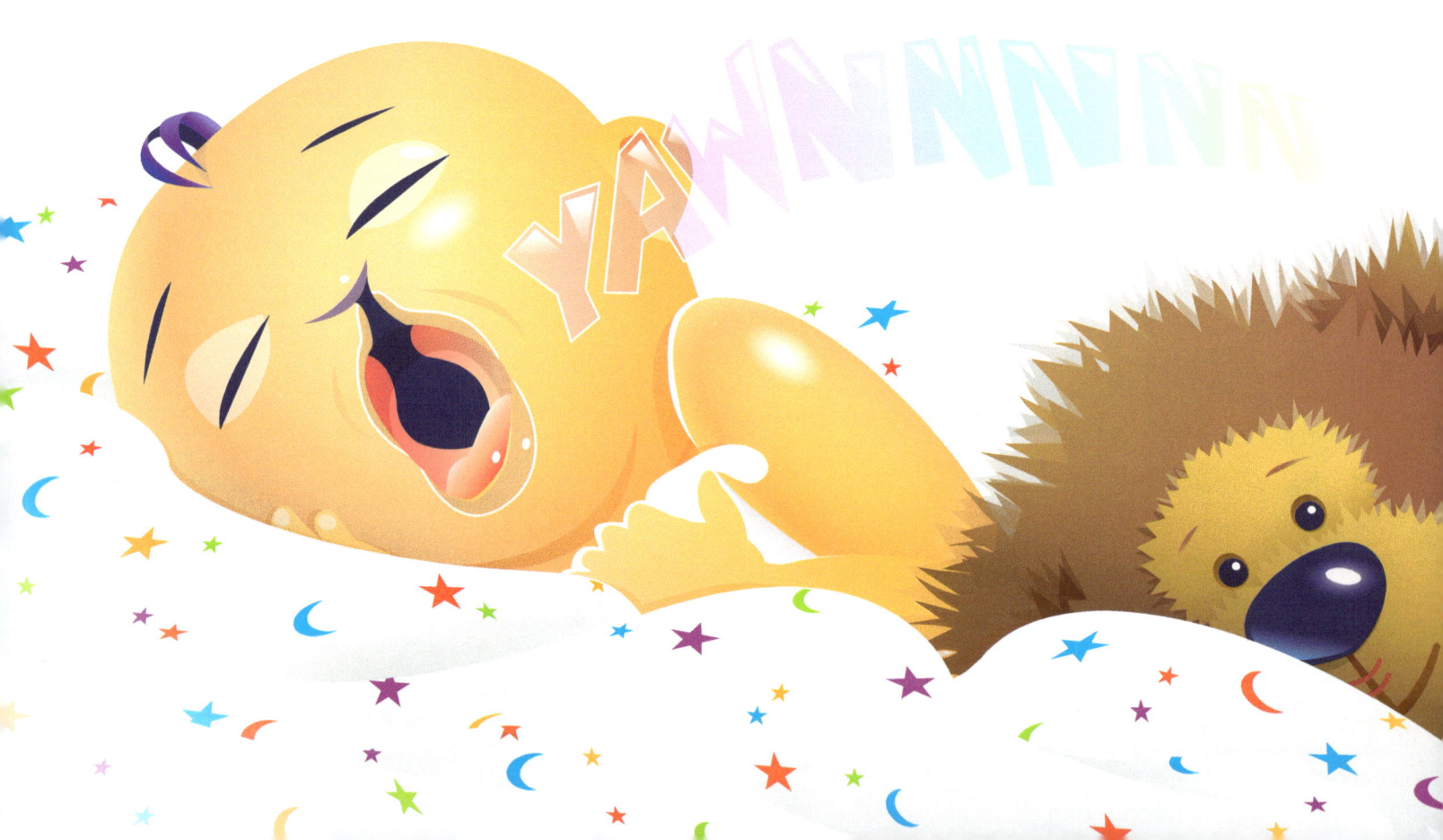

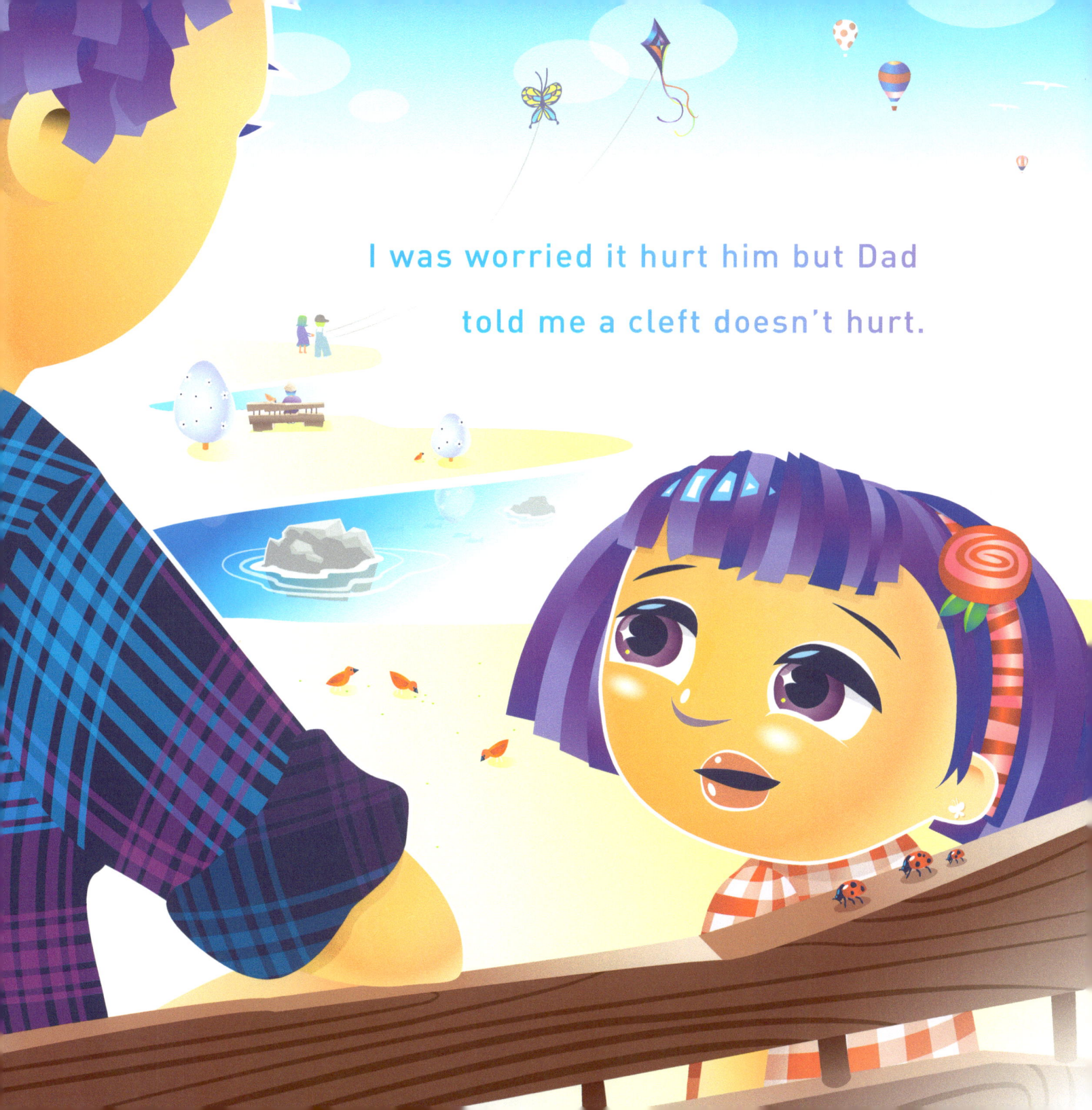

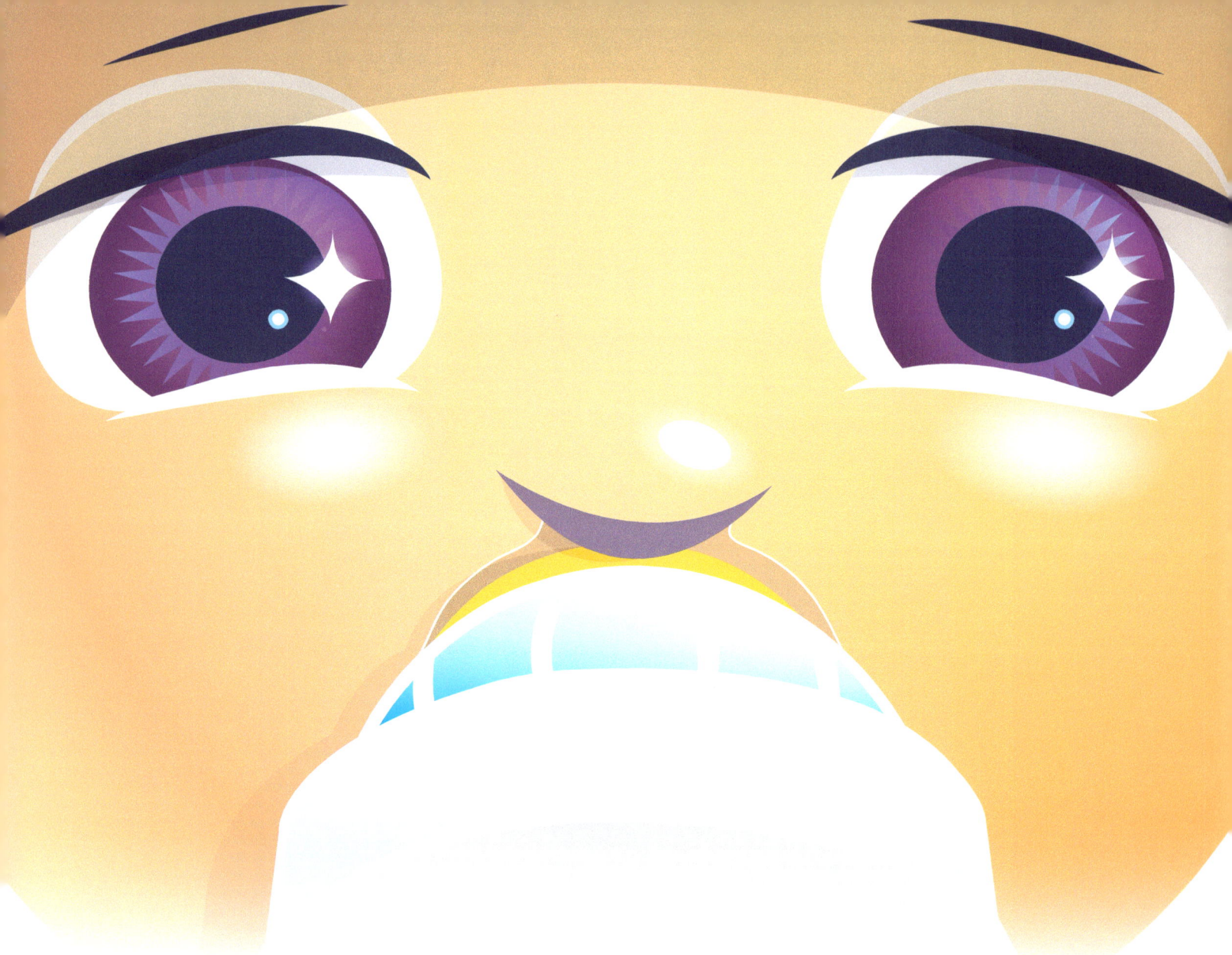

Jack has special bottles to help him drink.

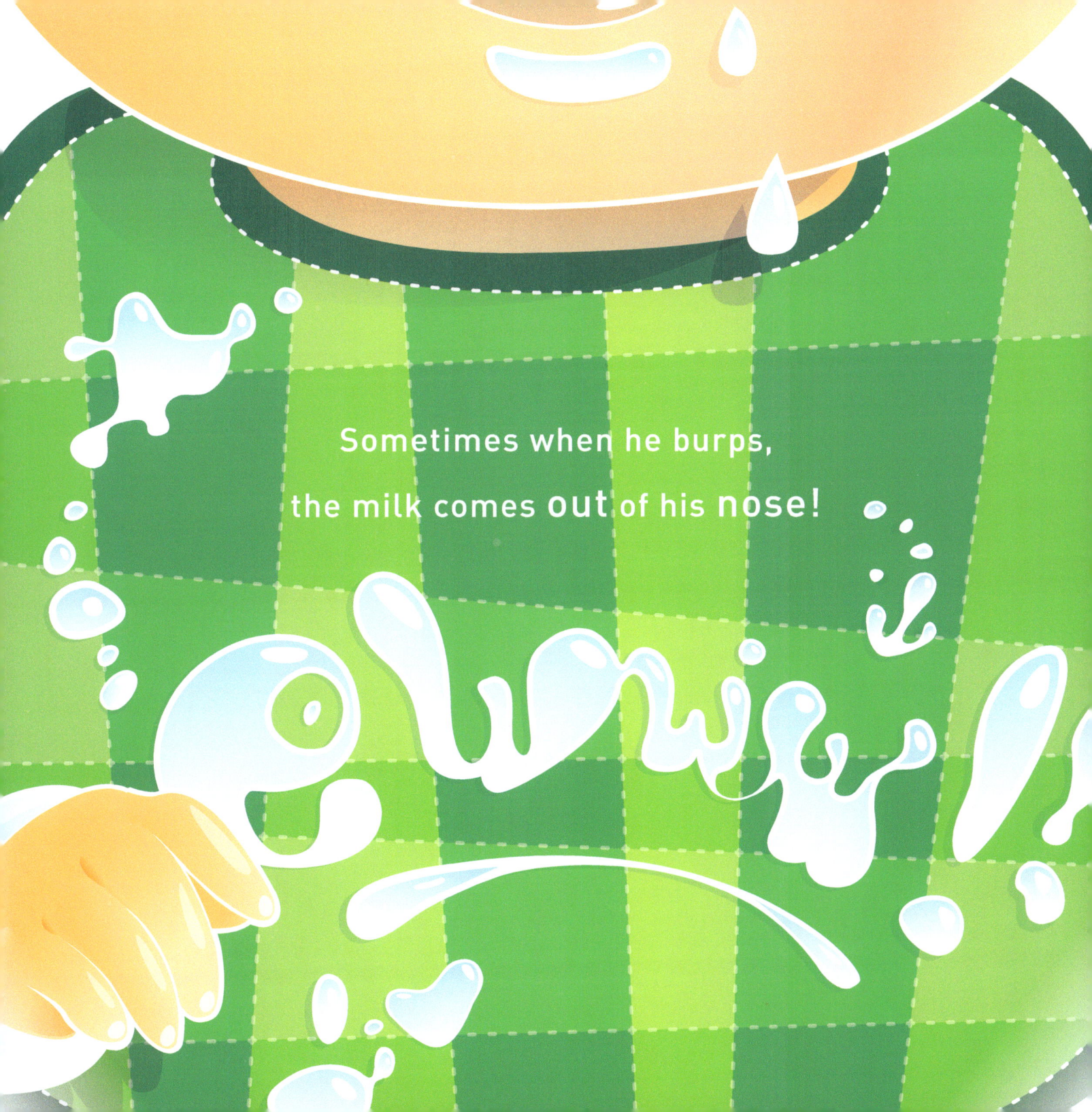

Sometimes when he burps,
the milk comes out of his nose!

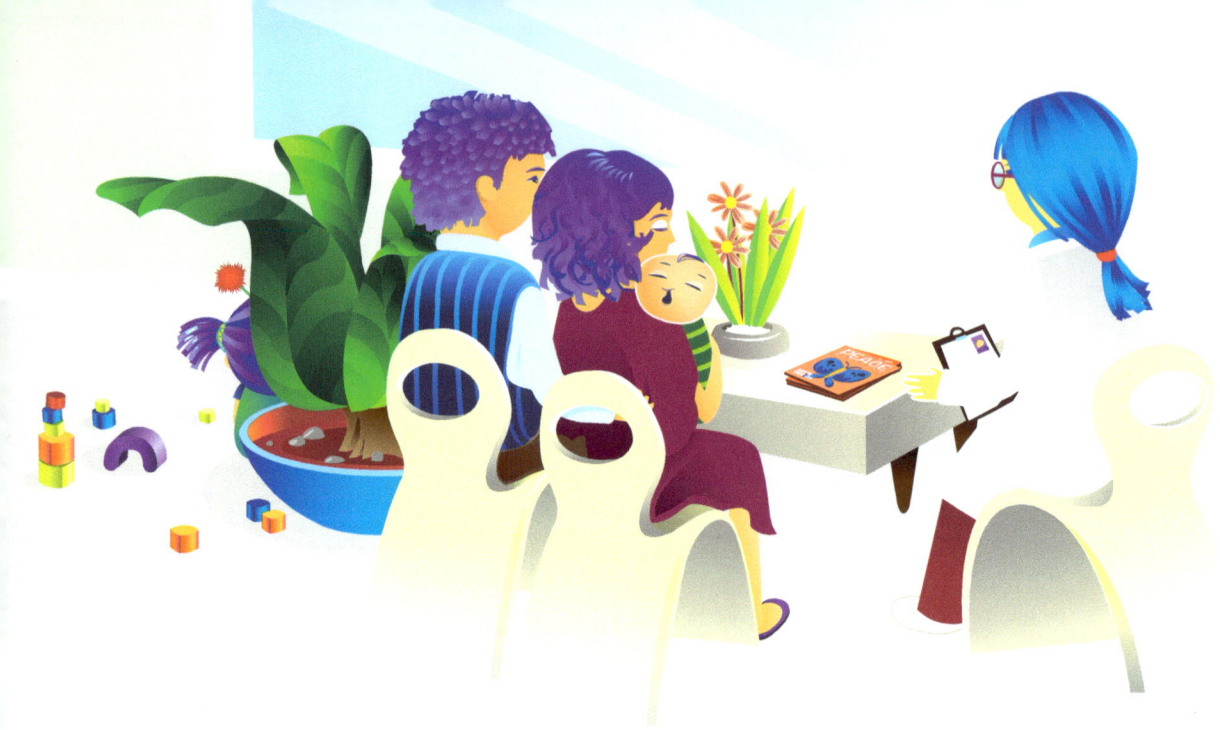

Today we went to the hospital to meet Jack's new doctor. Mom and Dad talked for a long time while I played with blocks!

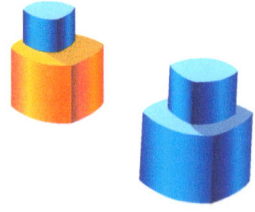
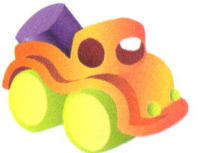

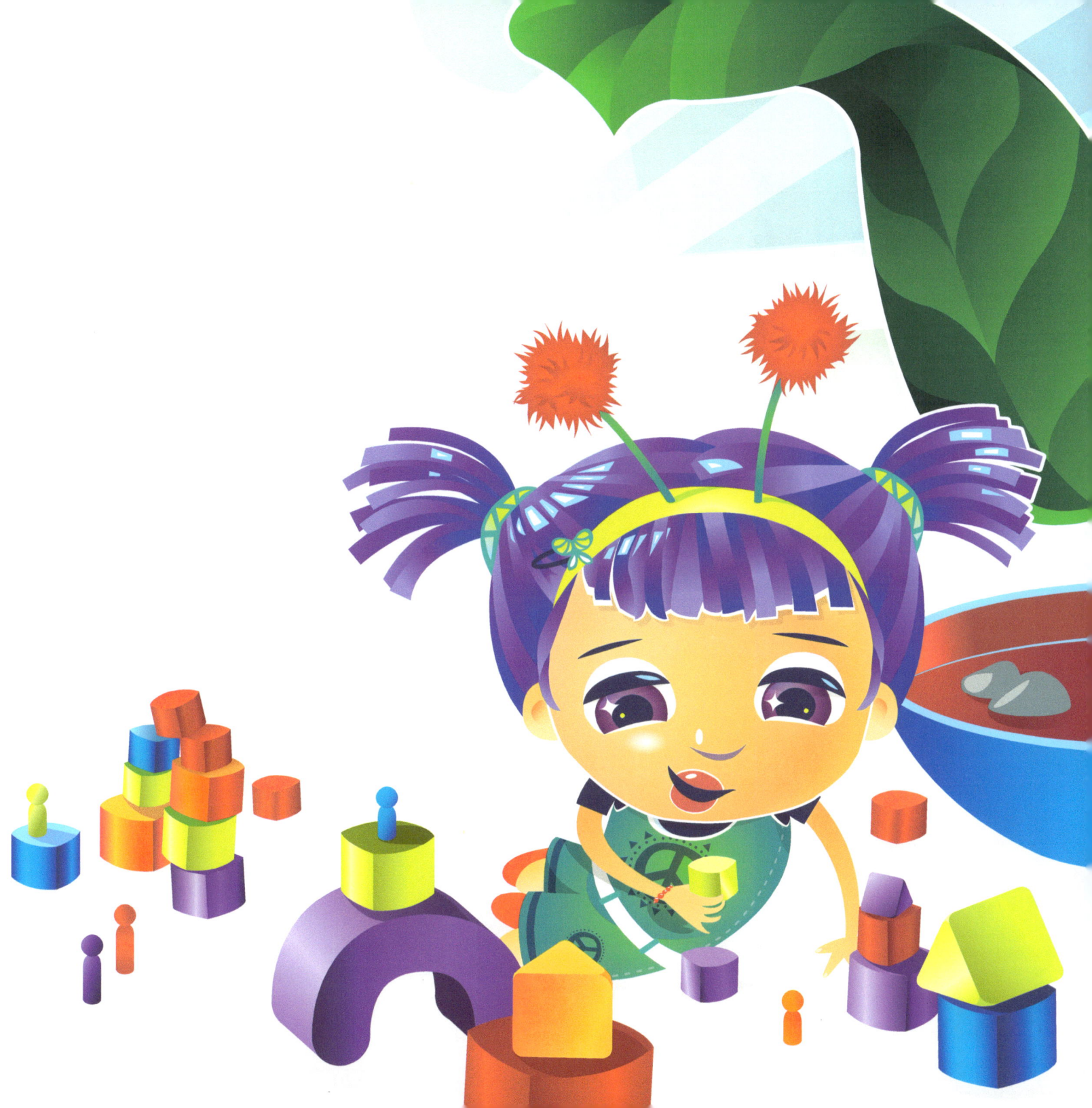

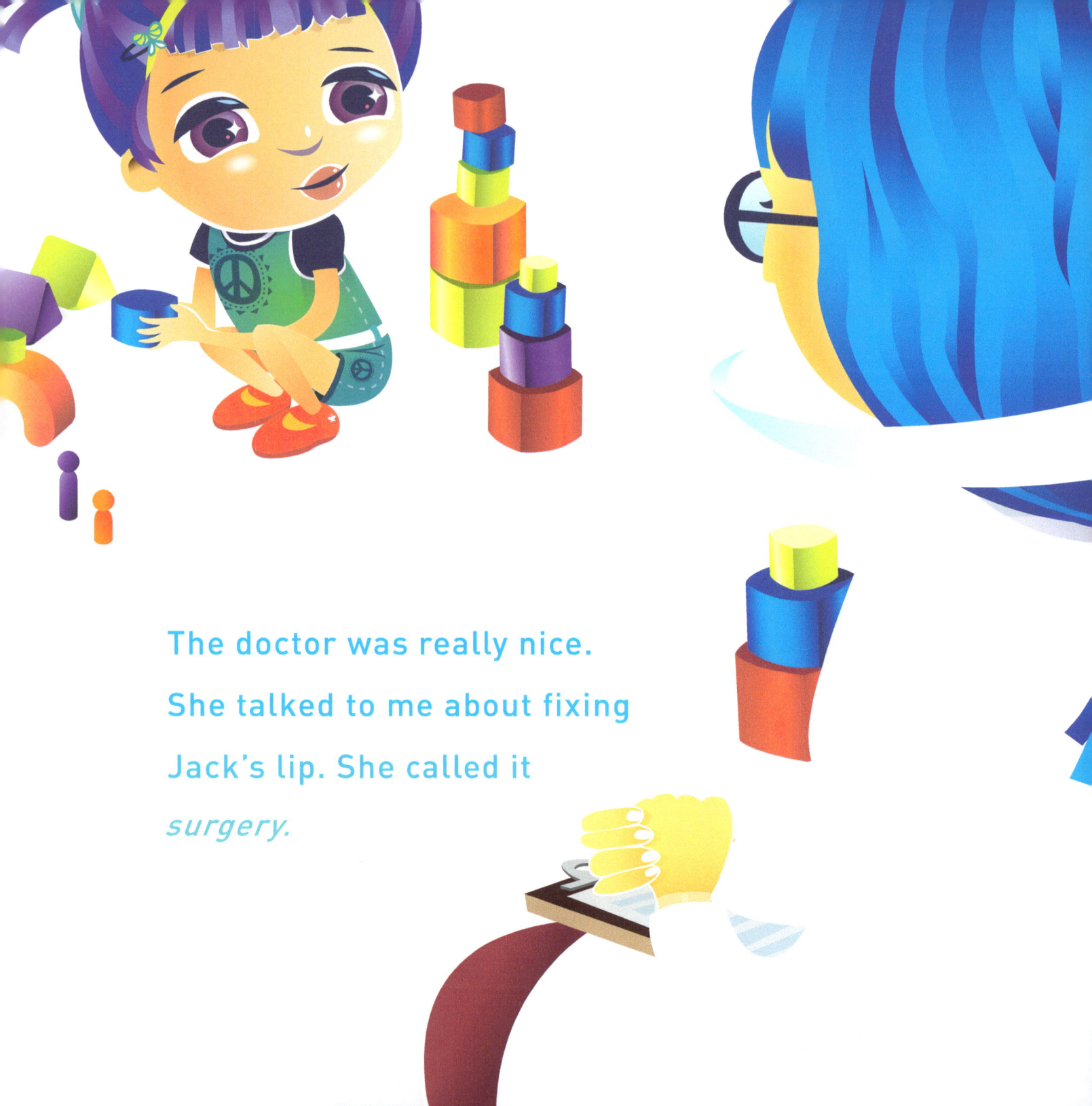

The doctor was really nice. She talked to me about fixing Jack's lip. She called it *surgery.*

I'll fix Jack's lip.
It won't hurt him.
Doctors will give him
medicine to help
him sleep until the
surgery is over.

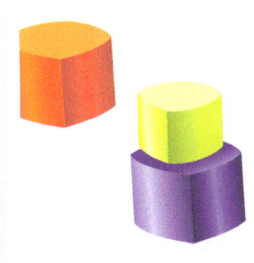
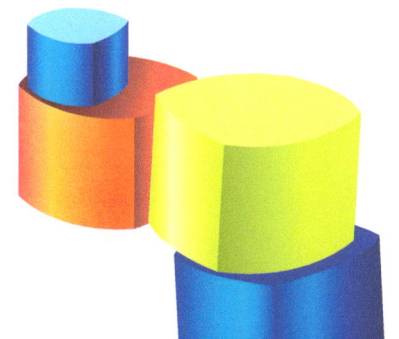

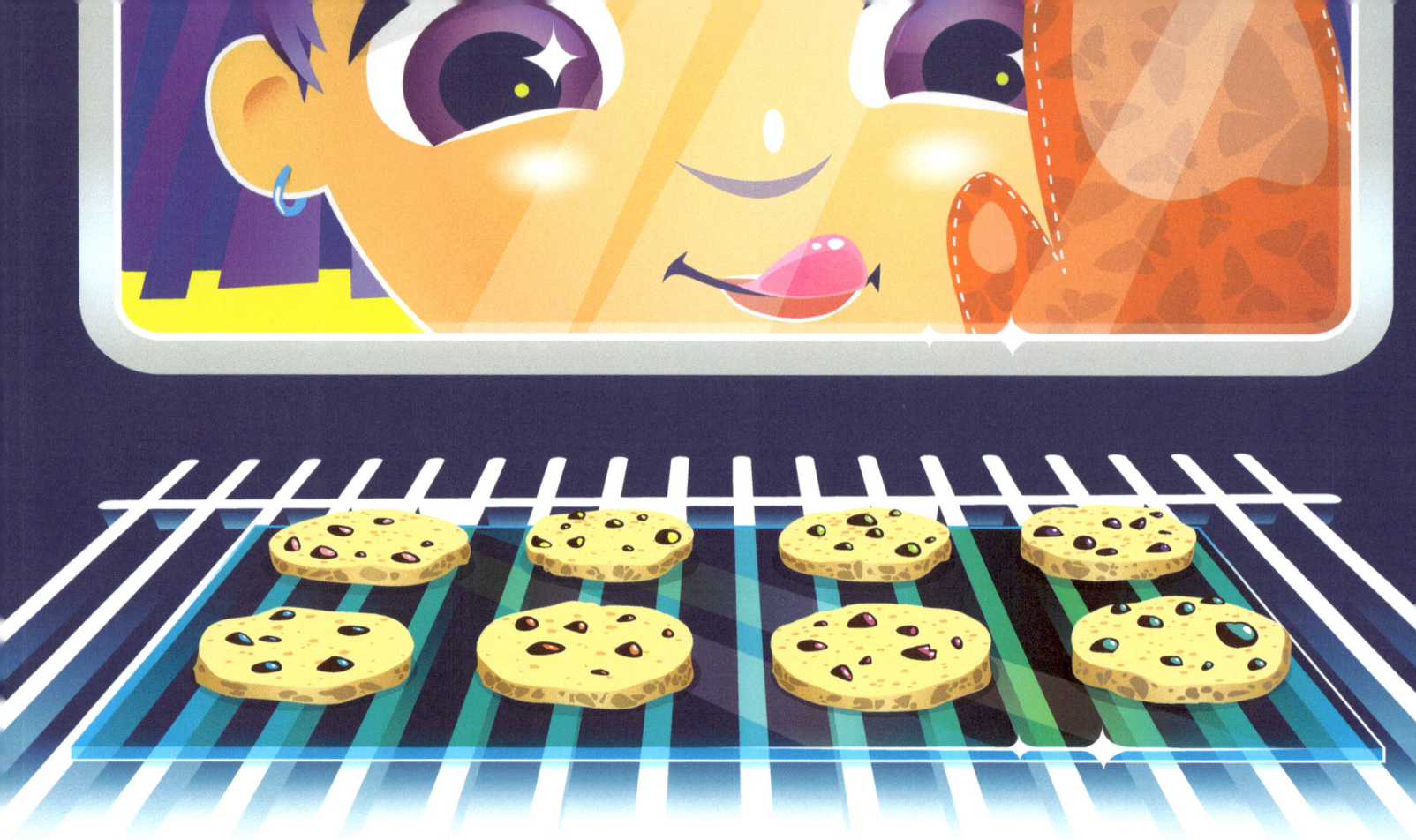

Mom and Dad took Jack to the hospital.
They stayed with him so he wouldn't be scared.
Grandma and Grandpa came to my house.
We baked cookies!

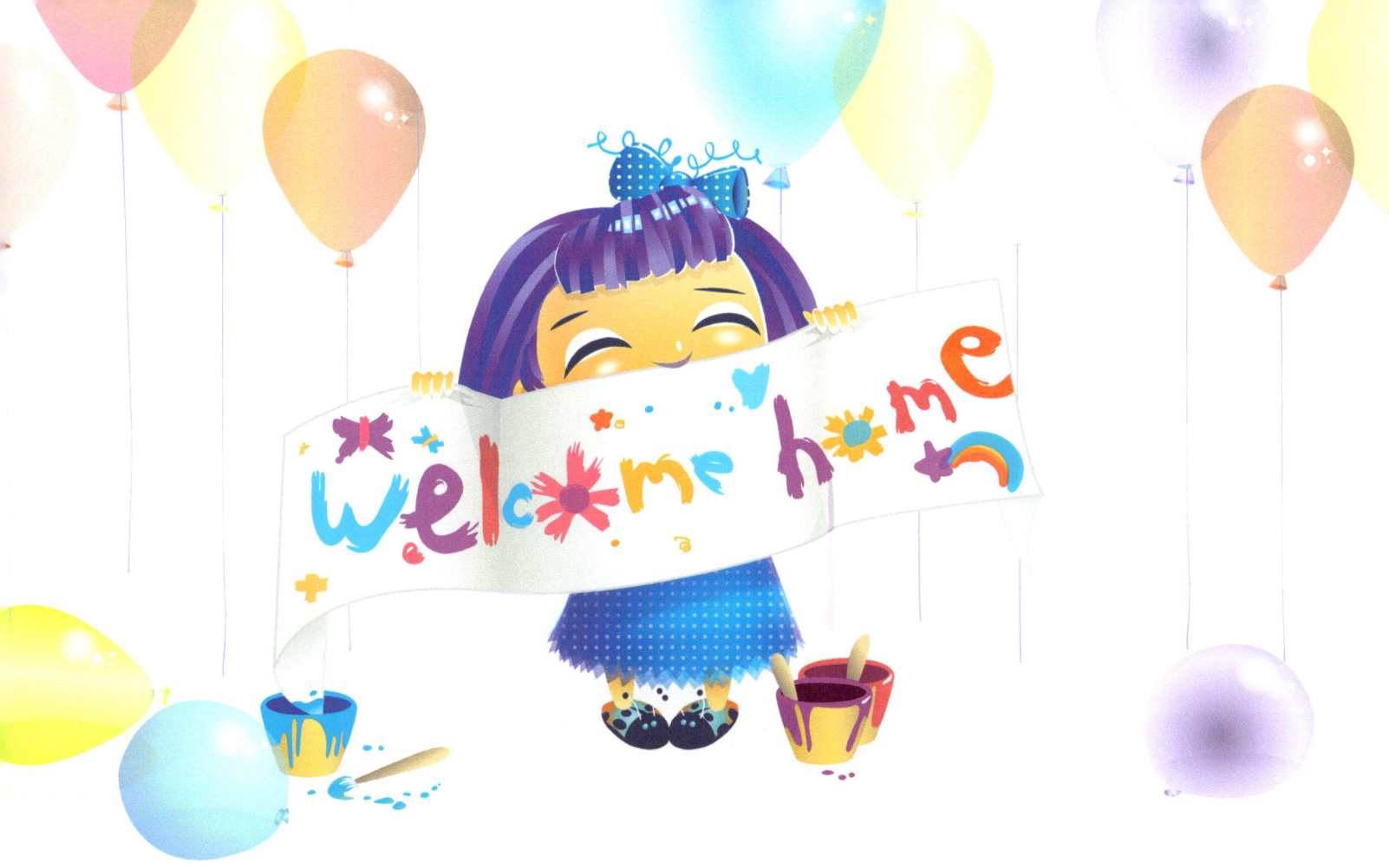

I could hardly wait for them to come home.

Look at the banner I made for Jack!

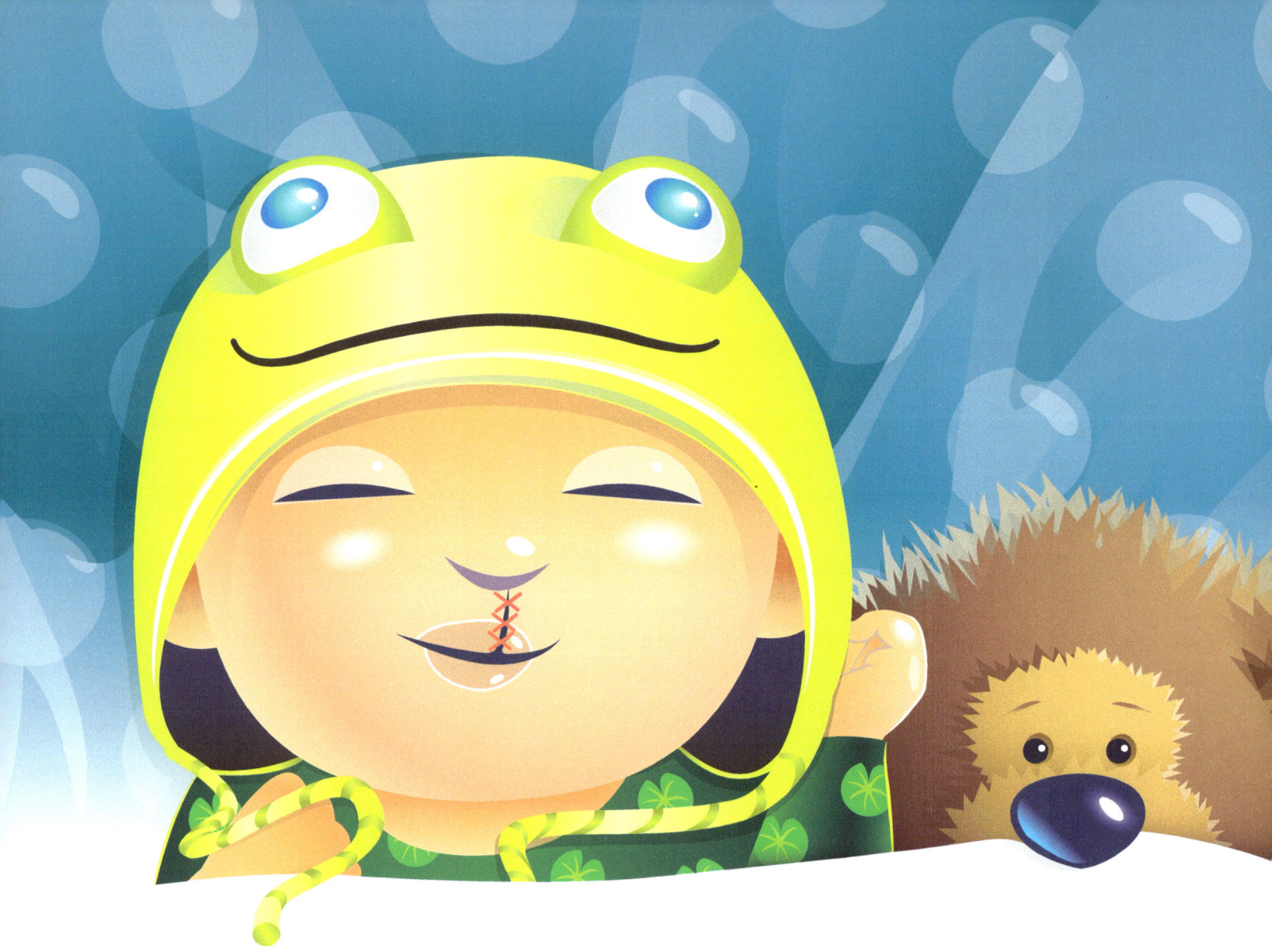

After the surgery, Jack's lip looked a lot like mine! He still has the cleft palate. Mom says he'll need another surgery to fix it when he is bigger.

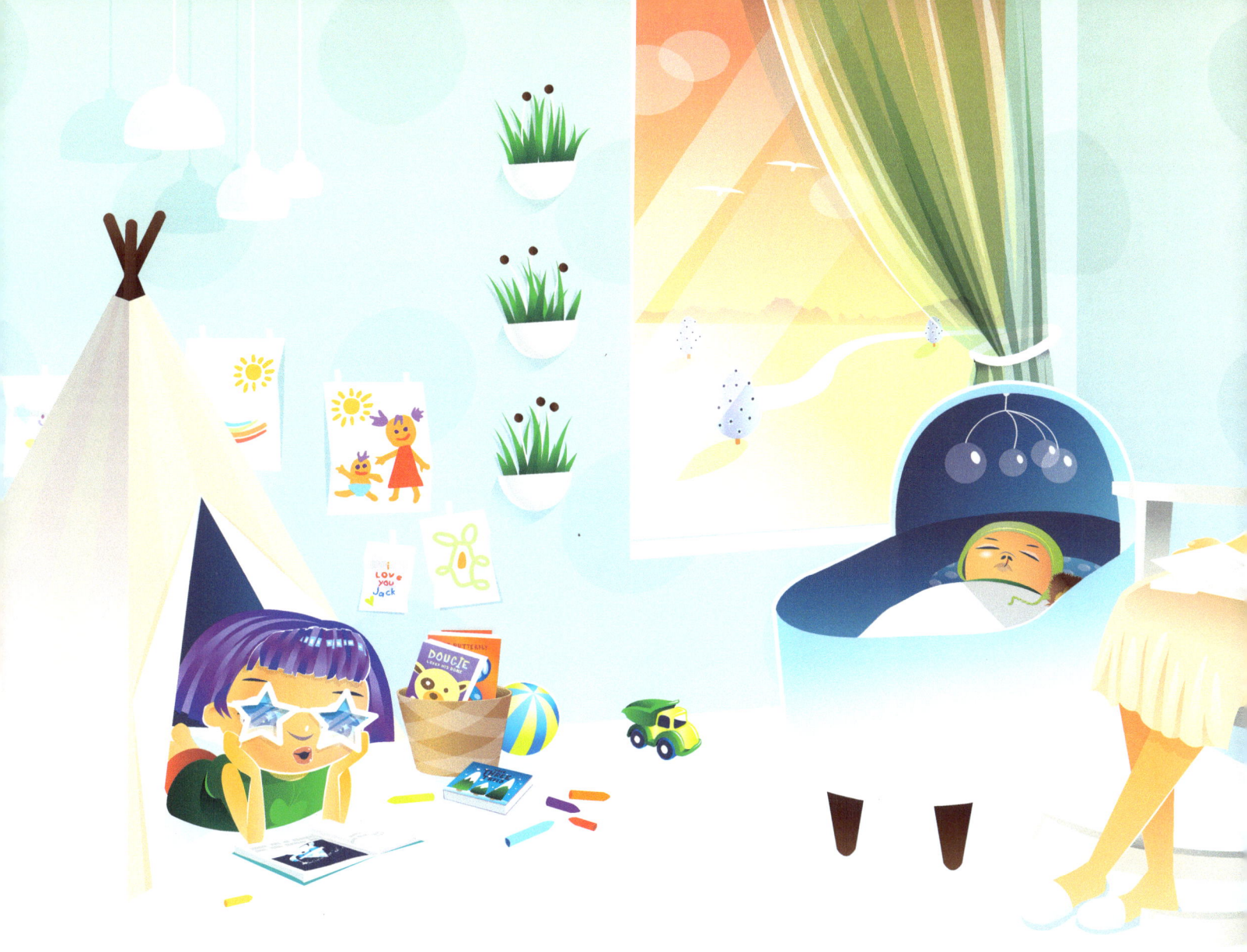

I had to be careful around Jack for
A WHOLE WEEK after he came home.

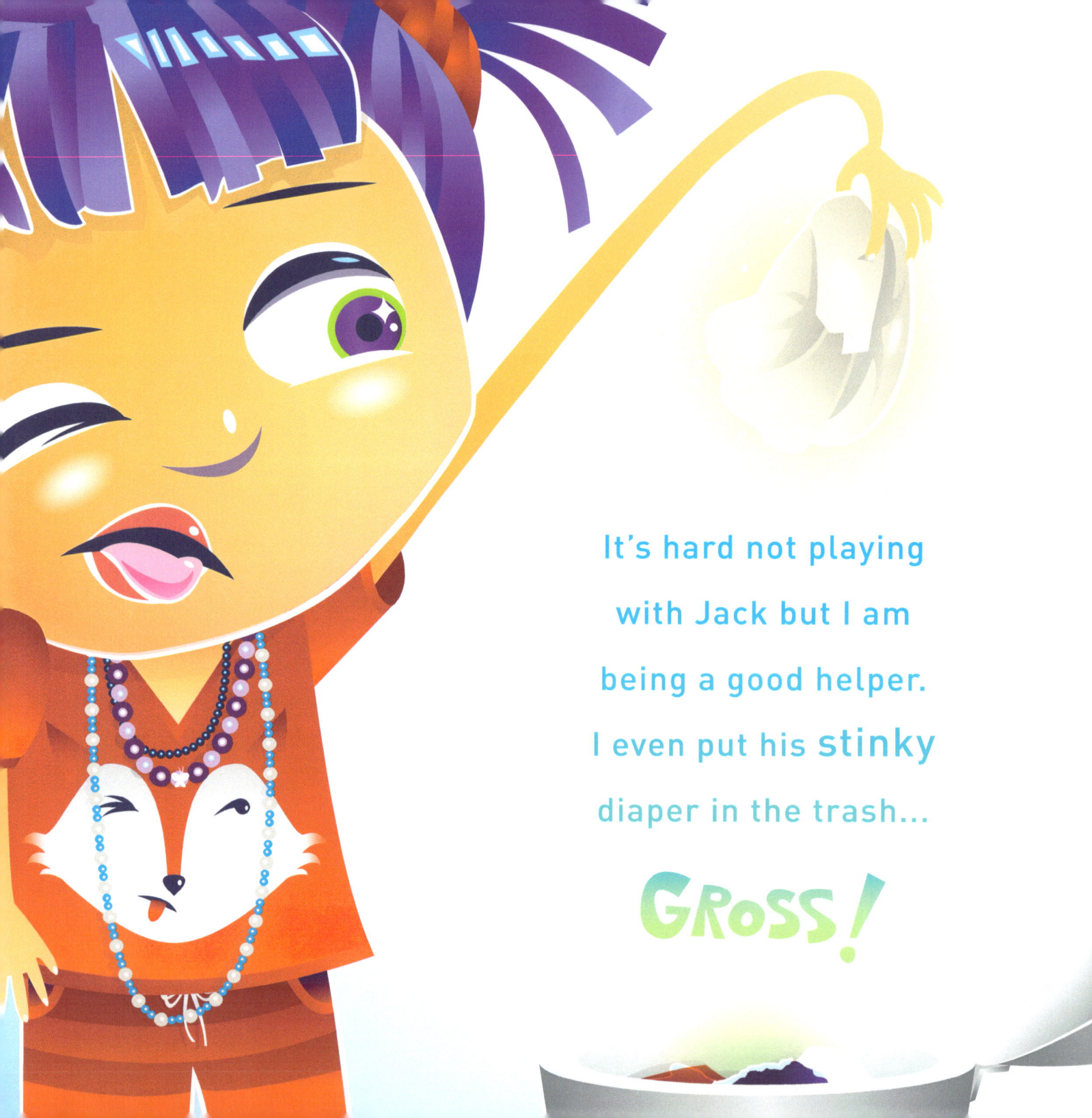

It's hard not playing with Jack but I am being a good helper. I even put his **stinky** diaper in the trash...

GROSS!

I have been such a good big sister that Dad surprised me with a trip to the zoo! The monkeys **really** made me laugh!

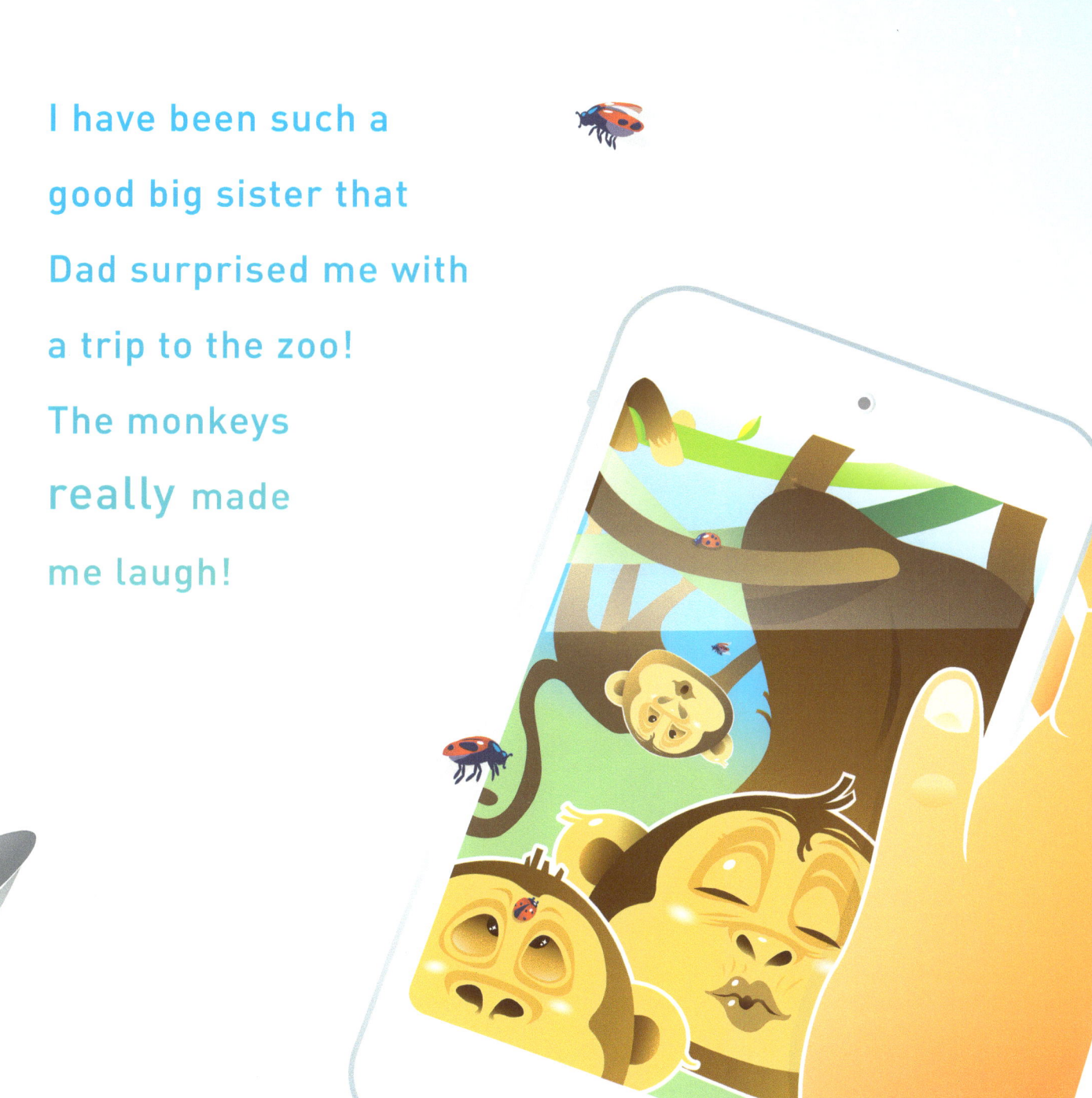

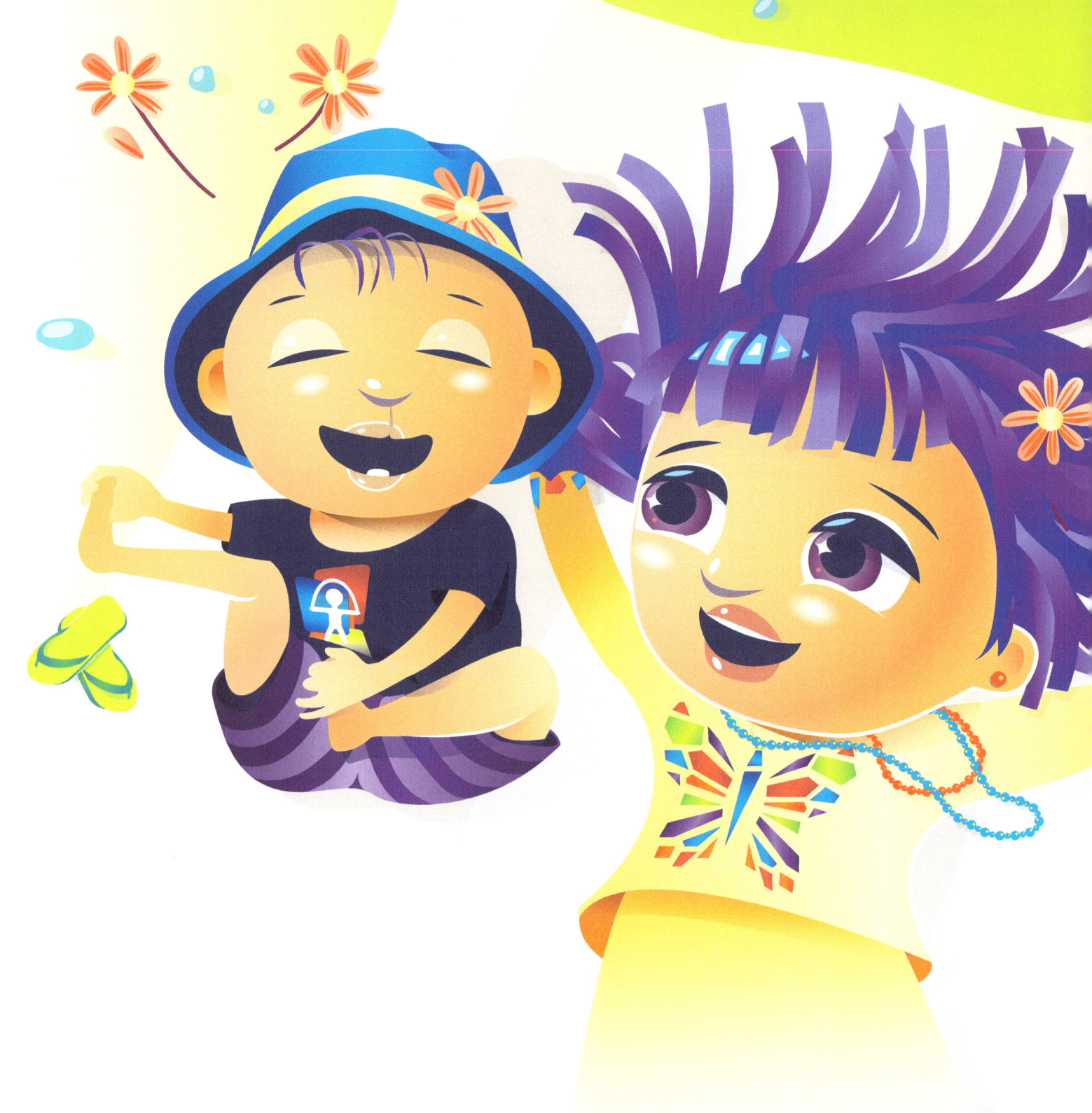

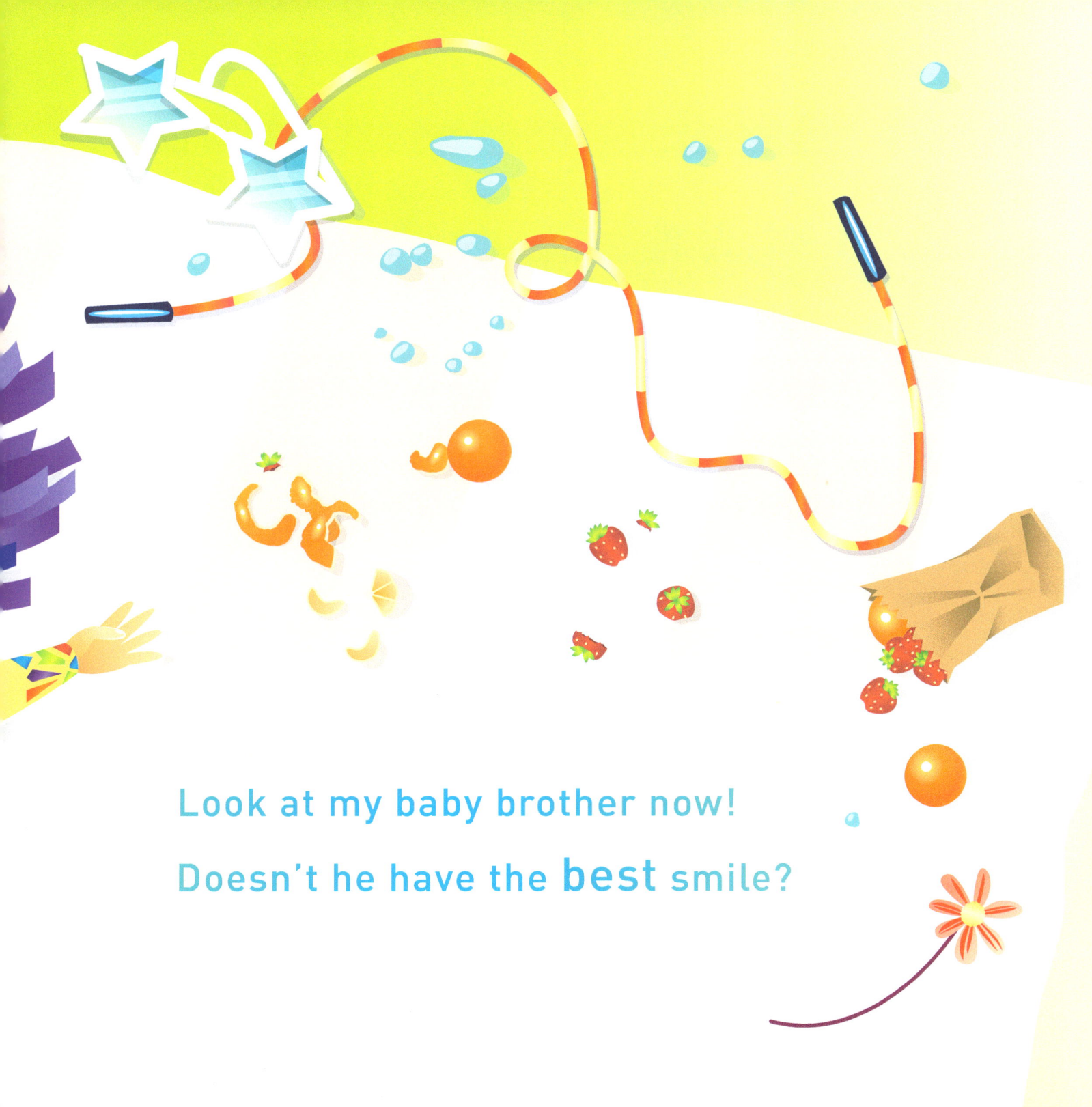

Look at my baby brother now!

Doesn't he have the **best** smile?

INFORMATION FOR FAMILIES

What is Cleft Lip/Cleft Palate?
Cleft lip and/or palate is one of the most common birth differences in babies. One of every 600 children is born in the United States with a cleft. A cleft lip is an opening or separation in the lip. It may occur on either side or on both sides of the lip. Having a cleft lip also changes the look of the nose. A cleft palate is an opening in the roof of the mouth. A cleft happens during the first few months of pregnancy. The reasons are often unknown but is usually not something a parent has done wrong. There are many possible causes for clefts, and research is helping us learn more.

Can A Cleft Be Fixed?
Cleft lip is usually repaired with surgery in the first few months of life. Cleft palate can be fixed some months later, often around one year of age. The timing of surgery depends on your baby's health and the doctor who does the surgery. You should feel comfortable with your surgeon and not be afraid to ask lots of questions.

Will My Baby Be Able to Eat?
If your baby has cleft lip alone, feeding is not usually a problem. A baby with a cleft palate may have more problems with feeding and need special bottles and nipples. A specialist who works with a cleft team will be able to help you with feeding your baby. It is important to seek help as soon as possible after your baby is born.

Will My Baby Have Problems Learning to Talk?
Speech is usually not a problem if your baby has only cleft lip. If your child has cleft palate, after it is repaired, a speech therapist will carefully follow your child's speech. Some children born with cleft palate will need speech therapy. A few may need another surgery to help their speech.

Will a Cleft Change My Baby's Teeth?
Cleft lip may affect just the lip or it may go into the gum. A baby whose cleft goes into the top gum will probably need dental specialists. All children need to see a dentist to keep teeth clean and healthy.

How Can I Make Sure My Baby Is Getting the Right Care?
The best care for your baby is with an experienced cleft team. Providers on this multidisciplinary team work together in a coordinated manner. Your child may need to see many specialists as he or she grows up. These may include plastic surgery, speech therapy, ear examinations, hearing testing, and dental care including orthodontic treatment. The cleft team will work with you to make sure that, together, you make the best choices for your child.

For more information about cleft lip and palate, contact:
Cleft Palate Foundation
800.24.CLEFT
info@cleftline.org
www.cleftline.org

Center for Craniofacial Care
www.craniofacial.vcu.edu
804.828.3042

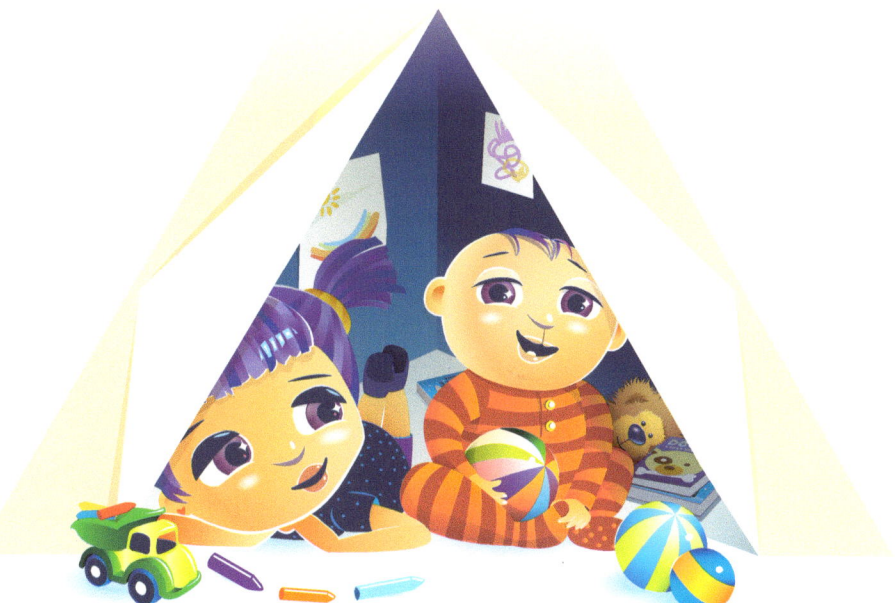

ABOUT THE AUTHORS

Ruth M. Trivelpiece, MEd, CCC-SLP is a speech/language pathologist who serves as the Program Coordinator for the Center for Craniofacial Care & Vascular Birthmark Clinic at Children's Hospital of Richmond at Virginia Commonwealth University. An active member of the American Cleft Palate-Craniofacial Association, she has served for over 30 years working with children & families with craniofacial differences. Ruth is nationally recognized for her expertise on issues related to craniofacial speech & feeding management, the importance of team care, & health literacy.

Suzanne N. West, MSN, MSLS, BS, RN is a nurse at VCU Health Systems. She earned her MS in Library Science from Clarion University of Pennsylvania, Bachelor of Science in Nursing from Virginia Commonwealth University, & her Master of Science with a concentration in family nurse practitioner from Virginia Commonwealth University. She enjoys using her combined educational experience to promote health information literacy & health condition education.

Jennifer L. Rhodes, MD, FAAP, FACS is Associate Professor of Surgery & Pediatrics at the Virginia Commonwealth University School of Medicine. Dr. Rhodes is a board certified plastic surgeon at Children's Hospital of Richmond at VCU where she serves as the medical director for the Center for Craniofacial Care & Vascular Birthmark Clinic. She received her medical degree from the University of Pennsylvania. She completed a general Surgery residency at St. Vincent's Hospital & Medical Center, a plastic surgery residency at Montefiore Medical Center, and craniofacial fellowship training with Jeffrey Fearon, MD, at The Craniofacial Center in Dallas, Texas. She is a member of the American Society of Plastic Surgeons, the International Society of Craniofacial Surgery, The American Cleft Palate-Craniofacial Association, & the American Academy of Pediatrics. Dr. Rhodes is committed to caring for children & families, focusing on all aspects of care related to their conditions as needed throughout their lives.

Brooke D. N. Fetissoff is an artist of various mediums. To be a part of this book has been a dream come true. Her next big dreams are to illustrate other educational children's books & to help actualize world peace.

www.ingramcontent.com/pod-product-compliance
Lightning Source LLC
Chambersburg PA
CBHW051819210526
45473CB00005B/1658